Pocket Guide to Malignant Melanoma

Pocket Guide to Malignant Melanoma

John Buchan

MBChB, MRCGP, DRCOG, DFFP, DPD
General Practitioner and Clinical Assistant
  in Dermatology
Rhayader
Powys
Wales

Dafydd Lloyd Roberts

MB, BS, FRCP (London)
Consultant Dermatologist
Swansea NHS Trust
Wales

Foreword by
Professor John Hawk

MD, FRCP
Head of Photobiology Department
Guy's, King's & St. Thomas School of Medicine
And Honorary Consultant Dermatologist
Guy's & St. Thomas NHS Trust
London, UK

**Blackwell
Science**

© 2000 by
Blackwell Science Ltd
Editorial Offices:
Osney Mead, Oxford OX2 0EL
25 John Street, London WC1N 2BL
23 Ainslie Place, Edinburgh EH3 6AJ
350 Main Street, Malden
  MA 02148 5018, USA
54 University Street, Carlton
  Victoria 3053, Australia
10, rue Casimir Delavigne
  75006 Paris, France

Other Editorial Offices:
Blackwell Wissenschafts-Verlag GmbH
Kurfürstendamm 57
10707 Berlin, Germany

Blackwell Science KK
MG Kodenmacho Building
7–10 Kodenmacho Nihombashi
Chuo-ku, Tokyo 104, Japan

The right of the Author to be
identified as the Author of this Work
has been asserted in accordance
with the Copyright, Designs and
Patents Act 1988.

First published 2000

Set by Graphicraft Limited, Hong Kong
Printed and bound in Spain by
Hostench s.a., Barcelona.

The Blackwell Science logo is a
trade mark of Blackwell Science Ltd,
registered at the United Kingdom
Trade Marks Registry

DISTRIBUTORS

Marston Book Services Ltd
PO Box 269
Abingdon, Oxon OX14 4YN
(*Orders*: Tel: 01235 465500
          Fax: 01235 465555)

USA
Blackwell Science, Inc.
Commerce Place
350 Main Street
Malden, MA 02148 5018
(*Orders*: Tel: 800 759 6102
          781 388 8250
          Fax: 781 388 8255)

Canada
Login Brothers Book Company
324 Saulteaux Crescent
Winnipeg, Manitoba R3J 3T2
(*Orders*: Tel: 204 837-2987)

Australia
Blackwell Science Pty Ltd
54 University Street
Carlton, Victoria 3053
(*Orders*: Tel: 3 9347 0300
          Fax: 3 9347 5001)

A catalogue record for this title
is available from the British Library

ISBN 0632054212

Library of Congress
Cataloging-in-publication Data

Buchan, John, MBChB, MRCPG, DRCOG,
DFFP, DPD.
  Pocket guide to melanoma /
John Buchan, Dafydd Lloyd Roberts.
    p. cm.
    Includes index.
    ISBN 0-632-05421-2
    1. Melanoma–Handbooks, manuals, etc.
I. Roberts, Dafydd Lloyd. II. Title.
RC280.M37 B83 2000
616.99'477—dc21   99–053650

For further information on
Blackwell Science, visit our website:
www.blackwell-science.com

Contents

Foreword

Malignant melanoma is one of the most aggressive cancers, killing some 1500 people in the United Kingdom every year, a rate which has been doubling about every 10–12 years, probably because of population lifestyle changes leading to much more frequent and intense sun exposure episodes. The good things about melanoma, however, if such things are possible, are that it can to a large extent be avoided if care is taken in the sun from a young age, and that it is also virtually completely curable if caught early. What has therefore been needed has been a compact, easy to read and readily understandable book which clearly explains this and everything else of note about melanoma so that the reader becomes easily well-informed without the need to spend huge amounts of time trawling through multiple pages of complex information. Fortunately Drs John Buchan and Dafydd Roberts, the former a principal in general practice in Powys, Wales, a clinical assistant in dermatology, a founder member of the Primary Care Dermatology Society and a member of the UK Skin Cancer Working Party, and the second a leading consultant dermatologist in the Swansea NHS Trust, Chairman of the UK Skin Cancer Working Party and an author of many papers on skin cancer, have realised this and produced exactly the concise, easily comprehensible book needed for everybody involved in melanoma at all levels. I now strongly recommend the result — readers will not be disappointed.

Professor John Hawk

Preface

The latter half of the twentieth century has witnessed a global rise in the incidence of malignant melanoma. Education campaigns and increased public awareness have led to many more patients with pigmented lesions seeking advice. This book provides an illustrated, up-to-date overview of the epidemiology, aetiology, diagnosis, surgical and second-line management, histopathology, follow-up and prevention of malignant melanoma. The book is aimed at family physicians, dermatologists in training, junior doctors, specialist dermatology nurses, senior medical students and other professionals involved in skin cancer prevention.

1 Epidemiology and Aetiology: Where, Who and Why

INTRODUCTION

Malignant melanoma is ten times more common today than 60 years ago. It is, in part, a preventable cancer and is curable if treated at an early stage. It will, however, prove fatal in around one in five cases. The death toll from melanoma is three times that of all other skin cancers combined and accounts for 90% of the skin cancer deaths in white people aged 15–50 years. Malignant melanoma should be a concern for us all.

EPIDEMIOLOGY

Over the last three decades there has been a steep rise in the incidence of cutaneous malignant melanoma. Mortality too has risen, but less rapidly. Reliable data from many countries show this to be a world-wide phenomenon. The highest recorded incidence is found in the residents of Queensland, Australia, now closely followed by the white population of South Africa. In many European Countries mortality and incidence is increasing at a rate of between 3% and 7% [1]. The disease is more common in northern Europe, with Norway having the highest incidence. In the USA the incidence of melanoma is increasing at a rate faster than that for any other cancer [2]. Similar rises have been reported in Canada and in Japan. In Scotland, where detailed records have been kept for some years, the incidence of melanoma in women appears to have stabilized, while mortality in younger women shows a downward trend [3]. There may be some levelling off of mortality in both the USA and Australia. There is, however, no room for complacency. The personal and social cost of malignant melanoma remains a cause for world-wide concern.

AETIOLOGY

Sun exposure

The main environmental risk factor for the development of cutaneous

1

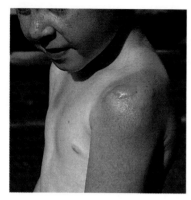

Fig. 1.1 Ouch!

malignant melanoma is exposure to solar ultraviolet (UV) radiation. Evidence for this has come from numerous epidemiological studies involving more than 10 000 patients [4]. The nature of the relationship is not entirely clear and involves a complex interplay between the type of sun exposure and certain individual, genetically determined characteristics. The relationship also varies with the type of melanoma (See Chapter 2). Superficial spreading and nodular melanomas do not always occur on the sites of greatest sun exposure. The less common lentigo maligna melanoma develops most frequently on the faces of those who have had a high lifetime sun exposure.

The intermittent exposure of fair skin to strong sunlight is an important factor in the development of melanoma. A smaller but still significant risk exists for overall lifetime sun exposure. More people are taking holidays in sunny resorts and a suntan is still perceived by many as desirable. A history of frequent sunburn increases the risk of melanoma, a fact that applies to both childhood and adult life. The risk related to sunburn and sun exposure may be greater in childhood (Fig. 1.1). This is supported by studies of emigrants from the UK to Australia and New Zealand. Those who arrived after the age of 15 have a lower incidence of melanoma than do children born in these countries.

Table1.1
Fitzpatrick skin types.

Type 1	White skin, never tans, always burns
Type 2	White skin, burns initially, tans with difficulty
Type 3	White skin, tans easily, burns rarely
Type 4	White skin, never burns, always tans. Mediterranean type
Type 5	Brown skin
Type 6	Black skin

There is evidence that people of the same skin type have a higher risk of melanoma the closer they live to the equator. The incidence is 10–12 times higher in white skinned than in black skinned races living in the same environment.

Skin specialists around the world have expressed concern that further depletion of the ozone layer, with the subsequent loss of protection from solar UV radiation, will result in even higher levels of malignant melanoma and other skin cancers.

Skin type

An individual's skin type and response to sun exposure are important in determining the likelihood of developing melanoma. Table 1.1 shows Fitzpatrick skin types.

Skin type is fixed for life and those with skin types 1 and 2 are at greater risk [5]. Large numbers of freckles, red or blonde hair, or blue eyes also increase the risk. For example, having red hair as opposed to dark hair more than doubles one's chances of developing melanoma [6]. Malignant melanoma is very rare in those with skin types 5 and 6.

World-wide studies have confirmed that people with larger numbers of common melanocytic naevi ('moles') are at greater risk of developing malignant melanoma [7]. The presence of atypical naevi (dysplastic naevi or atypical mole syndrome) is an even stronger risk factor. Sun exposure appears to increase the numbers of both common and atypical melanocytic naevi.

Children, families, pregnancy and the oral contraceptive

Melanoma is rare in prepubertal children. About 50% of childhood melanomas arise from giant congenital naevi, although the risk of an individual lesion developing malignant change has been calculated at approximately 4%. The even rarer condition of xeroderma pigmentosa is also an established risk factor. If the two preceding conditions are excluded, work from Australia has shown that the development of melanoma in childhood has similar epidemiological characteristics to adulthood.

Both a family history and a personal history of previous malignant melanoma increase the individual risk. Not only do children inherit the genetic susceptibility but often they adopt the same sunbathing habits as their parents.

In Western Europe the female to male ratio is almost 2 : 1. This is not so marked in other parts of the world.

Melanomas that arise during pregnancy are often thicker than tumours arising in non-pregnant women of childbearing age but may not carry a less favourable prognosis. Therapeutic abortion does not improve the cure rate and subsequent pregnancies are at no greater risk. There is no evidence linking the oral contraceptive to malignant melanoma [8].

Other UV sources

Artificial sources of ultraviolet radiation are a cause for concern. Modern sun beds emit UVA, which is responsible at least for photo-ageing of the skin. A UVA induced tan has only a sun protection factor (SPF) of 2 and may give the recipient a false sense of security. It is often those with an inability to tan who are most anxious to use sun beds. Older sunlamps that emit both UVA and UVB should be discarded.

Preliminary follow up of neonates treated with phototherapy for hyperbilirubinemia (jaundice) so far have shown no significant risk of developing malignant melanoma, however the median follow-up time was only 18 years [9].

There is a small increased incidence of melanoma found in psoriatic patients who have received 250 or more PUVA treatments (photochemotherapy with oral psoralen and UVA). It is rare for patients with psoriasis to receive such a large number of treatments [10].

Social factors

Both higher income and higher education appear in some way to be linked to melanoma. It is not clear whether this is merely a reflection of lifestyle.

There is no association between the development of melanoma and smoking, alcohol intake or diet.

REFERENCES

1 Osterlind A. Epidemiology on malignant melanoma in Europe. *Acta Oncol* 1992; **31**: 8: 903–8.

2 Koh HK, Geller AC. Melanoma control in the United States: current status. *Recent Results in Cancer Res* 1995; **139**: 215–24.

3 MacKie RM, Hole D, Hunter JA *et al.* Cutaneous malignant melanoma in Scotland: incidence, survival and mortality 1979–94. *BMJ* 1997; **315**: 7116: 1117–21.

4 Elwood JM. Melanoma and sun exposure. *Seminars Oncol* 1996; **236**: 650–66.

5 Lu H, Edwards C, Gaskell S, Pearse A, Marks R. Melanin content and distribution in the surface corneocyte with skin phototypes. *Br J Dermatol* 1996; **135**: 2: 263–7.

6 Bliss JM, Ford D, Swerdlow AJ *et al.* Risk of cutaneous melanoma associated with pigmentation characteristics and freckling: systematic overview of 10 case-control studies. *Int J Cancer* 1995; **62**: 4: 367–76.

7 Bataille V, Grulich A, Sasieni P *et al.* The association between naevi and melanoma in populations with different levels of sun exposure: a joint case-control study of melanoma in the UK and Australia. *Br J Cancer* 1998; **77**: 3: 505–10.

8 Holly EA, Cress RD, Ahn DK. Cutaneous melanoma in women III. Reproductive factors and oral contraceptive use. *Am J Epidemiol* 1995; **141**: 10: 943–50.

9 Berg P, Lindelof B. Is phototherapy in neonates a risk factor for malignant melanoma development? *Arch Pediatrics Adolescent Med* 1997; **151**: 12: 1185–7.

10 Stern RS, Nichols KT, Vakeva LH. Malignant melanoma in patients treated for psoriasis with methoxsalen (psoralen) and ultraviolet A radiation (PUVA). *New England J Med* 1997; **336**: 15: 1041–5.

2 Diagnosis: Suspicions, Scoring and Special Diagnostic Aids

Early diagnosis, immediate referral and appropriate surgical intervention are of paramount importance in reducing the mortality from malignant melanoma. If correctly managed, very thin, superficial lesions have an excellent prognosis. The deeper a tumour invades, the more gloomy the outlook. For all professionals whose privilege it is to see and examine their fellow human beings, there is a responsibility to be on the lookout for any suspicious pigmented lesions. These professionals include doctors, nurses, physiotherapists, chiropodists, dentists and opticians. Public awareness campaigns should not only encourage safer attitudes towards the sun but also advise on appropriate self-examination and self-referral of possible melanomas.

WHAT MAKES A LESION 'SUSPICIOUS'?

It is difficult for the nonspecialist to acquire for themselves sufficient expertise in the diagnosis of melanoma. In some parts of the world specific pigmented lesion clinics have been set up, but not every patient has access to such a specialized service. Inappropriate referral of common benign lesions can quickly overwhelm these clinics. To address this dilemma, clinicians have sought to devise sensitive screening tests for melanomas. Two diagnostic aids are currently in common usage.

1 MacKie's revised seven-point checklist (Table 2.1).

Pigmented lesions that display any of the three major signs should be considered for referral and the presence of any of the minor signs should further endorse this. Over 95% of all melanomas will show at least one major feature. Minor features are present in about 30–40%. Alternatively, a score of 2 points can be given for any major feature and 1 point for each minor feature present. Any lesion with one major feature or a score of 3 or more should be referred [1].

2 The ABCDE checklist (adapted from the American Cancer Society's ABCD checklist).

Table 2.1
MacKie's seven-point checklist.

Major features
Change in size
Change in colour
Change in shape

Minor features
Diameter equal to or more than 7 mm
Sensory changes
Ooze/crusting/bleeding
Inflammation

The US system of ABCDE (A for asymmetry, B for border irregularity, C for colour irregularity, D for diameter greater than 6 mm and E for elevation) is easy to remember and works well for established melanomas, although it does not reflect change occurring in a pigmented lesion. Changing features are important diagnostic indicators of early melanoma [2].

HISTORY

A history should be obtained from every patient presenting with a suspicious pigmented lesion. This history should include the patient's age, occupation and degree of sun exposure, particularly episodes of sunburn. Inquiry should be made into whether or not the patient comes from a 'moley' family and if there is a personal or family history of melanoma or mole removal. A note should be made of how long the lesion has been present and what prompted consultation. Has there been any recent change in size, colour or shape either noted by the patient or by anyone else? Has the lesion become inflamed, bled, oozed or itched?

EXAMINATION

The lesion should be examined in good light and its position on the body recorded. The largest diameter should be measured and particular note made of its shape, looking especially for asymmetry and an irregular border. Variation in the pigment should also be recorded—is the pigment unevenly distributed, does the colour vary? Are there any signs of weeping, crusting, bleeding or inflammation? Are the regional lymph nodes enlarged? The rest of the skin should be examined and skin type, hair colour, the presence of freckles and number of moles or atypical naevi noted.

From the history and examination the lesion can be given a score—either from the seven-point checklist or the ABCDE—and referral considered. Irrespective of scoring systems, if there remains clinical doubt as to the diagnosis of the lesion, then a further opinion should be obtained.

TYPES OF MELANOMA

There are four main types of melanomas:

1. superficial spreading melanoma;
2. nodular melanoma;
3. lentigo maligna melanoma;
4. acral lentiginous melanoma.

Superficial spreading melanoma

Over half of the melanomas presenting on white skinned people are superficial spreading melanomas. They are more frequently found in women than men. The commonest sites are the lower legs of women and the back in men. The latter is not easy to self examine and hence there may be a delay in seeking help. Superficial spreading melanomas usually present in mid-life but the age of presentation is declining and 18% of melanoma cases now occur in people aged between 15 and 39 years.

Typically, lesions are variably pigmented with an irregular border and are slightly raised (Fig. 2.1). Normal skin markings may be lost and there may be evidence of inflammation. The period of superficial growth, during which time the tumour spreads laterally, may last several months. Growth and partial regression during this period may alter the appearance with central areas of pigment loss (Fig. 2.2). The development of thickening or nodules indicates that the tumour has entered the vertical invasive growth phase with rapidly worsening prognosis. Oozing, bleeding or crusting occurs later if the lesion is ignored. Although superficial spreading melanomas may arise in normal skin, they more frequently arise in a pre-existing mole.

Nodular melanoma

Nodular malignant melanomas are more common in men. They tend to present later in life, being more common in the fifth and sixth decades.

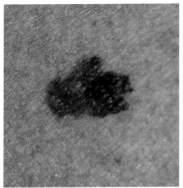

Fig. 2.1 Superficial spreading melanoma.

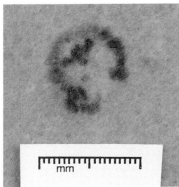

Fig. 2.2 Superficial spreading melanoma with central pigment loss (courtesy of Dr J Evans, Derriford Hospital, Plymouth).

They comprise 20–25% of all melanomas. The favoured sites are the trunk, head and neck. Unlike superficial spreading melanomas there is no lateral growth phase, the tumour invades vertically from the outset, it grows rapidly and, as a consequence, the tumour carries a poorer prognosis. Nodular melanomas present as elevated dome-shaped or even tag-like lesions (Fig. 2.3). The colour varies from reddish through to brown or black. A common presentation is of a red raised central lesion with a peripheral brown ring or crescent of melanin. Bleeding is frequently an early sign and the tumour may be easily confused with a vascular lesion. Amelanotic melanomas are rare (1–2% of all melanomas). Most are nodular and careful examination will often reveal a rim of pigment. Other types of melanoma may develop nodules as part of their later development. The absence of invasive melanoma cells in the adjacent epidermis distinguishes nodular melanomas from other forms of melanoma.

Lentigo maligna melanoma

Lentigo maligna melanomas are usually found in those over the age of 60 who have long histories of chronic sun exposure. There is frequently a background of extensive sun damaged skin. The commonest site is the face although about 10% are found on other exposed sites such as the

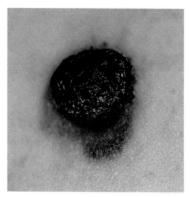

Fig. 2.3 Nodular melanoma.

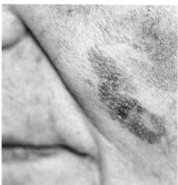

Fig. 2.4 Lentigo maligna.

hand and leg. There is a long pre-invasive phase that may extend over several years. During this phase the lesion appears as a very slowly growing flat, brown, irregular 'tea-stain' on the skin (lentigo maligna, Hutchinson's melanotic freckle or premalignant melanosis of Dubreuilh). Loss of skin markings and a very smooth, matt surface are useful diagnostic features (Fig. 2.4). Serial photographs may demonstrate expansion of the lesion. (Tip—ask the patient for old photographs). Initially the colour distribution is even but, with time, the pigmentation becomes irregular with areas of dark brown, blue or black; red or purple hues are less frequently noted. The development of an elevated nodule indicates a shift into the vertical invasive growth phase of a lentigo maligna melanoma (Fig. 2.5). If neglected, bleeding, oozing or even ulceration may occur.

Acral lentiginous melanoma

Acral lentiginous melanomas are found on the palms, soles and around the nail bed, usually of the big toe. They comprise approximately 10% of melanomas in the white skinned population with the sole of the foot being the most favoured site. About half of the melanomas arising on the palms and soles are of this variety. In Japan, about 50% of all melanomas are acral lentiginous melanomas. These lesions are characterized by a large flat pigmented area around a focus of melanoma that appears raised and may bleed or ooze. Patients are often unaware of lesions on the sole of the foot

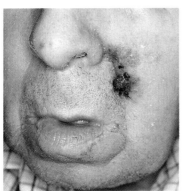

Fig. 2.5 Lentigo maligna melanoma.

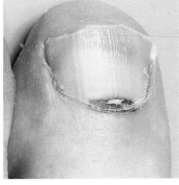

Fig. 2.6 Acral lentiginous melanoma. Note pigmentation proximal to the nail fold.

and delay seeking advice. Confusion with other lesions can delay diagnosis. Tumours around the nail bed are the most difficult to diagnose. A brown lesion below the nail may be mistaken for old blood. A very useful diagnostic sign (Hutchinson's sign) is brown/black pigmentation on the skin proximal to the nail (Fig. 2.6). Other presentations include longitudinal pigmentation, splitting, oozing, nail dystrophy and chronic paronychia. Destruction of the nail bed may be seen in advanced cases (Fig. 2.7).

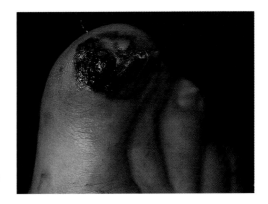

Fig. 2.7 Advanced acral lentiginous melanoma.

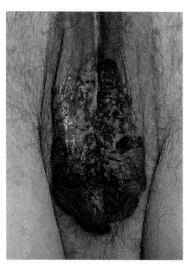

Fig. 2.8
Vulval melanoma.

LESS COMMON SITES AND PRESENTATIONS

Melanomas of mucosal sites share some of the characteristics of acral lentiginous melanomas. Irregular macular pigmentation of the oral cavity, vulvovaginal or rectal areas should be referred without delay (Fig. 2.8).

Areas of depigmentation may be seen around melanoma. The haloes are highly irregular whereas those around benign lesions tend to be even and symmetrical.

Biopsy of a suspicious nodule may reveal the presence of a secondary deposit. As well as a careful inspection of the skin, the mucous membranes and eyes should be thoroughly examined.

SPECIAL DIAGNOSTIC AIDS

Melanomas are not always easy to diagnose clinically. Good quality photos can be very useful in recording suspicious lesions or dysplastic naevi. Computerized image analyses have been developed to quantitatively measure shape and assess irregularity. Serial images are good at recording changing characteristics of lesions [3].

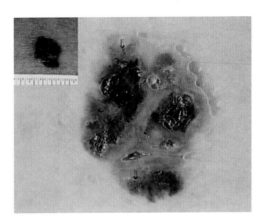

Fig. 2.9
Superficial spreading
melanoma viewed through
the dermatoscope, naked
eye appearance in corner
(courtesy of Heine
Optotechnik).

Skin surface microscopy relies on the recognition of pigmentary distribution patterns characteristic of melanoma, melanocytic naevi or other pigmented lesions. The dermatoscope, such as the DELTA 10 by Heine Optotechnik, offers affordable and portable skin surface microscopy for both the dermatologist and primary care physician. Resembling an otoscope, the dermatoscope gives approximately 10 × magnification with angled halogen illumination. The lesion is first moistened with suitable oil or disinfectant spray before being viewed through a glass disc attached to the underside of the dermatoscope (Fig. 2.9). With training and experience the use of the dermatoscope can increase clinical diagnostic accuracy of both benign and malignant lesions [4].

REFERENCES

1 Healsmith MF, Bourke JF, Osborne JE, Graham-Brown RAC. An evaluation of the revised seven-point checklist for the early diagnosis of cutaneous malignant melanoma. *Br J Dermatol* 1994; **130**: 48–50.
2 Whited JD, Grichnik JM. Does this patient have a mole or a melanoma? *JAMA* 1998; **279**: 9: 696–701.
3 Clardge E, Hall PN, Keefe M, Allen JP. Shape analysis for classification of malignant melanoma. *J Biomed Eng* 1992; **14**: 3: 229–34.
4 Nachbar F, Stolz W, Merkle T *et al*. The ABCD rule of dermatoscopy. High prospective value in the diagnosis of doubtful melanocytic skin lesions. *J Acad Dermatol* 1994; **30**: 4: 551–9.

FURTHER READING

1 MacKie RM. *Malignant Melanoma. A Guide to Early Diagnosis*. Glasgow
   University Department of Dermatology, 1989.
2 MacKie RM. Melanocytic naevi and malignant melanoma. In: Champion RH,
   Burton JL, Burns DA, Breathnach SM eds. *Textbook of Dermatology* 6th edn.
   Oxford: Blackwell Science, 1998, 1717–52.
3 Stolz W, Braun-Falco O, Bilek P, Landthaler M, Conetta AB. *Colour Atlas of
   Dermatoscopy*. Oxford: Blackwell Scientific Publications, 1994.

3 Differential Diagnosis: Moles and Much More

Fortunately the vast majority of pigmented lesions are not malignant melanoma. If the specialist services are not to be overwhelmed then it is important to be able to recognize and manage those common conditions that cause most diagnostic confusion. This chapter will consider both melanocytic lesions, where the pigment is predominantly melanin, and non-melanocytic lesions.

It must be stressed that all excised pigmented lesions should be sent for histological examination.

MELANOCYTIC NAEVI

We are all being encouraged to become 'mole watchers' and a request to 'check my moles' is increasingly common in primary care. The problem should be approached as outlined in Chapter 2, i.e. take a history, examine and apply the MacKie's seven point or ABCDE checklist. Reported recent change in the shape, size or colour of a mole should always be taken seriously and the possibility of malignant change considered. Knowing how the different types of melanocytic naevi present and evolve will aid the diagnosis and management.

Melanocytic naevi can be divided into congenital naevi, which are present at or around birth, and acquired naevi, which appear in later life.

Congenital melanocytic naevi

About 1% of babies have congenital naevi. These are divided into small (less than 1.5 cm in diameter), intermediate (1.5–20 cm in diameter) and giant (over 20 cm in diameter). Most are small. All tend to grow with the child and, over the years, become raised, darker and may develop a few coarse terminal hairs (Fig. 3.1). The very rare giant lesions carry approximately a 4–5% risk of malignant transformation with about half doing so before puberty (Fig. 3.2). Because of this, and also the understandable parental distress generated by these lesions, early referral to a specialist centre is indicated [1]. Malignant change in small to

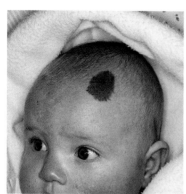

Fig. 3.1 Intermediate sized congenital naevus.

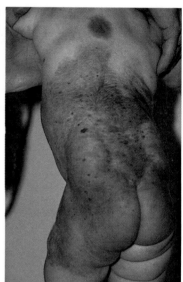

Fig. 3.2 Large congenital naevus.

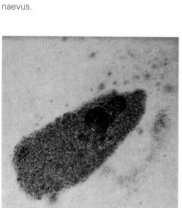

Fig. 3.3 Malignant change in a congenital naevus.

intermediate sized lesions is very uncommon and extremely rare before puberty. Parents should be advised to report any changing characteristics. Serial photographs can be a very useful aid (Fig. 3.3). Removal, if necessary, is best carried out between 10 and 13 years of age. Prophylactic excision of all congenital naevi, especially small lesions, is both impractical and unjustified in terms of melanoma risk [2].

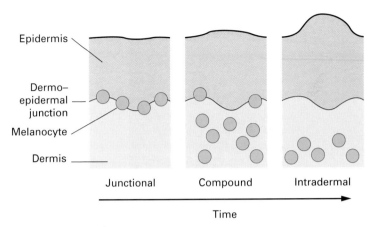

Epidermis			
Dermo–epidermal junction			
Melanocyte			
Dermis			
	Junctional	Compound	Intradermal

Time

Fig. 3.4 Naevus maturation.

Acquired melanocytic naevi

These are extremely common. On average, a white skinned young adult will have between 10 and 40 acquired melanocytic naevi. Many appear in infancy with a marked increase in the teenage years. Lesions may appear or become more noticeable during pregnancy. New melanocytic naevi otherwise seldom develop after early adulthood. Although their appearance may alter throughout life, there is a tendency towards spontaneous regression in old age. Acquired melanocytic naevi are rarely seen in the very elderly.

There are 3 main groups of acquired melanocytic naevi:

1 junctional.
2 compound.
3 intradermal.

These 3 types represent different stages of the same maturation process (Fig. 3.4).

As a naevus moves from junctional through compound to intradermal there is a migration of the proliferating melanocytes from the dermo–epidermal junction to within the dermis. These proliferating cells push up the overlying epidermis [3].

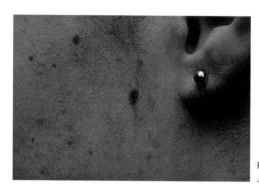

Fig. 3.5
Junctional naevus.

Junctional melanocytic naevi

These are the commonest naevi found in children. Lesions are usually flat, oval and light brown although there may be some variation in colour even within a single lesion (Fig. 3.5). Size varies from 1 mm to 1 cm or more. They feel like normal skin. Many progress with time into compound naevi, the exceptions being lesions on the palms, soles and genitalia which often retain their junctional form into adulthood.

Compound melanocytic naevi

In early to mid adult life this is the commonest type. These lesions are raised, a little larger and usually darker than junctional naevi (Fig. 3.6). They feel a little firmer than the surrounding skin. The slow process of

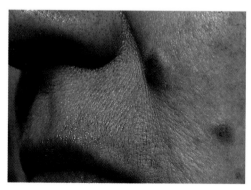

Fig. 3.6
Compound naevus.

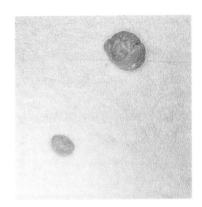

Fig. 3.7
Cerebriform compound
naevus.

development from junctional to compound is normal and does not
represent malignant change. The pigment is evenly distributed and the
lesions are usually smooth. Sometimes in larger lesions the epidermis is
thrown into folds giving a 'cauliflower' or cerebriform appearance (Fig. 3.7).

Intradermal naevi

These are found in older patients. They tend to be raised and less
pigmented than compound naevi, and are often pink or flesh coloured. Tiny
blood vessels may be visible on the surface of the lesion along with a few
coarse hairs. They are easily palpable. Intradermal naevi commonly occur on
the face (Fig. 3.8).

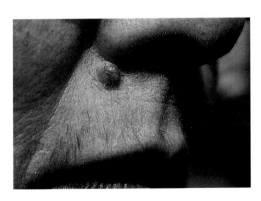

Fig. 3.8
Intradermal naevus.

Management of common acquired naevi

Intervention is not required in the great majority of cases. Suspected malignant change should prompt urgent referral to a specialist. All excised naevi, no matter how benign they may appear on clinical examination, should be sent for histological confirmation of diagnosis.

LESS COMMON ACQUIRED NAEVI

Spitz naevus

This lesion usually presents in childhood, often on the face, as a solitary pinkish red nodule that grows quite rapidly over a period of several months (Fig. 3.9). Because of their rapid growth they are frequently excised. Histologically they can resemble malignant melanoma hence their alternative but erroneous name of juvenile melanoma. They are, however, a variant of a compound naevus and are benign. If left then they become less red but more firm over the years.

Halo naevus (Sutton's naevus)

It is the area of depigmentation rather than the naevus itself that is the usual reason for consultation in Sutton's naevus (Fig. 3.10). Older children and teenagers are most commonly affected and the back and the shoulders the favoured sites. Halo naevi are often multiple and are more obvious on

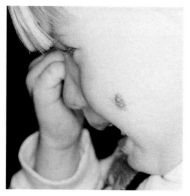

Fig. 3.9 Spitz naevus.

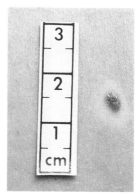

Fig. 3.10 Halo naevus.

tanned skin due to the lack of melanin production within the halo. The area of depigmentation is invariably symmetrical unlike that seen in malignant melanoma. Halo naevi are unusual in older patients and all patients over the age of 30 should be referred. Ultimately, both the central naevus and the halo will disappear although the latter may take years. No treatment is necessary but patients should be warned that the depigmented patch is much more prone to sunburn.

Blue naevi

Blue naevi present in early adulthood and, unlike other melanocytic naevi, persist for life. They are a uniform, dark blue–black in colour well demarcated, solitary and do not alter in appearance (Fig. 3.11). The commonest sites are on the face and backs of the hands. The potential for malignant change is very low and excision is usually for cosmetic reasons. If removed, the excision should extend to the subcutaneous fat as the aberrant melanocytes are situated deep within the dermis.

Dysplastic naevi

Some naevi have unusual features on clinical examination that makes them very difficult to differentiate from early melanoma. These dysplastic naevi are often larger (> 1 cm in diameter) and have an irregular border (Fig. 3.12). They may be inflamed or have an area of inflammation around them.

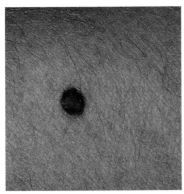

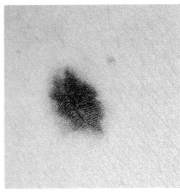

Fig. 3.11 Blue naevus.

Fig. 3.12 Dysplastic naevus.

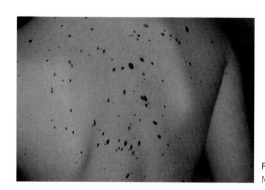

Fig. 3.13
Multiple dysplastic naevi.

Table 3.1
Classification of patients with multiple dysplastic naevi.

	Personal history of melanoma	Family history of multiple naevi	Family history of melanoma
A	No	No	No
B	No	Yes	No
C	Yes	No	No
D	Yes	Yes	Yes

The trunk is the most common site and lesions may be single or multiple (Fig. 3.13). Histological confirmation is usually necessary. It is important in assessing patients with dysplastic naevi to ascertain whether there is a personal or family history of melanoma or relatives with multiple naevi (Table 3.1).

Dysplastic naevi are at greater risk of developing into melanoma but the majority are stable and the relative risk depends on the classification. Patients with types A and B have a 4- and 8-fold increase in relative risk, respectively. For those with types C and D the increased risk may be several hundred-fold [4]. Patients with types C or D and their affected families are probably best kept under the surveillance of a specialist centre. Photographic records can be invaluable. Patients should be encouraged to report any change immediately and be particularly careful regarding sun exposure.

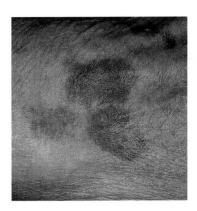

Fig. 3.14
Solar lentigo.

OTHER MELANOCYTIC LESIONS

Solar lentigo ('Senile' lentigo)

Solar lentigines appearing on the chronically sun exposed skin of older patients need to be differentiated from lentigo maligna melanoma. Lesions are often large, flat with a slightly irregular shape and of a uniform brown colour (Fig. 3.14). Solar lentigines may be seen in younger patients often following an acute episode of sunburn. Sun avoidance should be encouraged and some will spontaneously resolve. They can also be treated with cryotherapy.

NON-MELANOCYTIC LESIONS

Seborrhoeic keratosis (seborrhoeic wart, basal cell papilloma)

Seborrhoeic keratoses are very common benign epidermal tumours. Lesions are usually multiple but may be single (Fig. 3.15). They present from middle age onwards. Typically they have a 'stuck-on' appearance with a greasy, matt, crumbly surface speckled with keratin plugs ('currant bun' appearance, Fig. 3.16). The colour varies from tan through to dark brown or even black. Developed lesions are firm and discrete. In the classical form there is usually no doubt about the diagnosis but irritated lesions, developing lesions or lesions with marked variation in pigment may require biopsy. Flat lesions on the face can be confused with a lentigo melanoma—

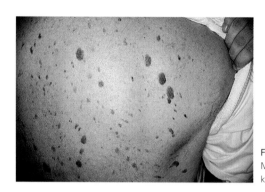

Fig. 3.15
Multiple seborrhoeic
keratoses.

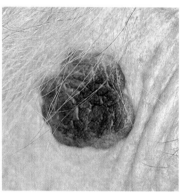

Fig. 3.16 Seborrhoeic keratosis.

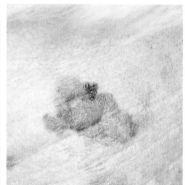

Fig. 3.17 Flat seborrhoeic keratosis on face.
A biopsy was required to confirm diagnosis.

a hand lens or skin surface microscopy can aid the diagnosis (Fig. 3.17).
Seborrhoeic keratoses can be removed easily by curettage and cautery or
cryotherapy. Lesions that catch on clothing or are particularly unsightly can
be dealt with in this way. The histology is diagnostic.

Dermatofibroma (histiocytoma, sclerosing angioma)

This benign dermal tumour usually occurs on the limbs and sometimes
appears to follow minor trauma (Fig. 3.18). The brown pigmentation is due
to the presence of iron and, less commonly, melanin. The lesion is quite

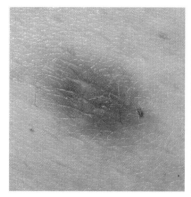

Fig. 3.18 Dermatofibroma.

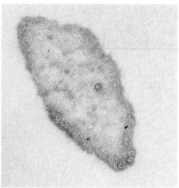

Fig. 3.19 Pigmented basal cell carcinoma.

firm and if squeezed from side to side the tethered overlying epidermis appears to dimple—a useful diagnostic sign. Excision is indicated if the diagnosis is in doubt.

Pigmented basal cell carcinoma

Occasionally, a basal cell carcinoma (rodent ulcer) will appear pigmented either due to the presence of melanin or due to bleeding within the tumour (Fig. 3.19). Close inspection will reveal the typical raised, rolled edge. Lesions are often translucent in part with fine telangiectasia. There may be central necrosis. Although they do not metastasize, they are locally destructive if ignored. Treatment is by excision with an appropriate margin. Radiotherapy is also effective. Small lesions may be treated with cryotherapy or curettage and cautery.

Pyogenic granuloma

A pyogenic granuloma may be easily confused with a nodular melanoma. They are, however, benign but rapidly growing vascular tumours provoked by minor trauma such as a prick from a sewing needle (Fig. 3.20). Children and younger adults are most often affected, with the hand being the commonest site. They grow rapidly over a period of a few weeks reaching a size of 5–10 mm. Lesions bleed easily and can vary in colour from bright red through to blue–black. Secondary infection is common. Spontaneous

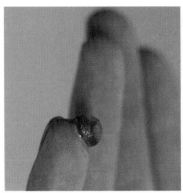

Fig. 3.20 Pyogenic granuloma.

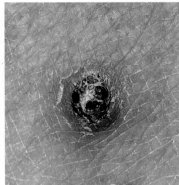

Fig. 3.21 Thrombosed angioma.

regression is rare and treatment is by curettage and cautery. Specimens should always be sent for histological confirmation.

Acquired angioma

A history of bleeding and a blue–black appearance due to thrombosis may lead to this lesion being confused with a nodular melanoma. Angiomas are usually raised and well demarcated from the surrounding skin (Fig. 3.21). It is sometimes possible to compress these lesions, for example with a microscope slide. They can be removed by excision with a narrow margin. This reduces the risk of further bleeding and allows histological confirmation of the diagnosis.

Talon noir

The pigmentation in this lesion is due to small blood vessel rupture with red blood cells leaking into the stratum corneum (Fig. 3.22). Lesions are usually found on the heel. There is often a history of trauma such as a sports injury or poorly fitting footwear. The skin markings are preserved and the pigment can be removed by gently paring away the horny layer confirming the diagnosis. No treatment is necessary.

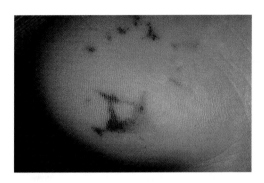

Fig. 3.22 Talon noir.

REFERENCES

1 Egan CL, Oliveria SA, Elenitsas R, Hanson J, Halpern AC. Cutaneous melanoma risk and phenotypic changes in large congenital nevi: a follow-up study of 46 patients. *J Am Acad Dermatol* 1998; **39**: 6: 923–32.

2 Chun K, Vazquez M, Sanchez JL. Malignant melanoma in children. *Int J Dermatol* 1993; **32:** 1: 41–3.

3 Anonymous. Consensus conference: Precursors to malignant melanoma. *JAMA* 1984; **251**: 14: 1864–6.

FURTHER READING

1 Barnhill RL. *Color Atlas and Synopsis of Benign and Malignant Pigmented Lesions*. New York. McGraw-Hill, 1995.

4 Histopathology and Natural History

Understanding the pathology report of a malignant melanoma is of fundamental importance, not only in confirming the diagnosis and type of lesion, but also in planning the definitive treatment and assessing prognosis. It is important to recognize the difficulties of diagnosing pigmented lesions histologically, and even expert pathologists sometimes disagree on borderline cases [1].

Malignant melanomas originate from the melanocytes of the basal layer of the epidermis. The essential histological feature of a malignant melanoma is that of abnormal melanocytes, usually with mitoses, involving both the epidermis and dermis. Superficial spreading malignant melanomas often have a period of time where they grow horizontally within the epidermis, and the whole of the epidermis may become infiltrated with large abnormal melanocytes (Pagetoid spread). Provided these stay within the epidermis they have no potential to produce metastases and are, therefore, a pre-invasive form of malignant melanoma. Once dermal invasion occurs, the lesion is then regarded as an invasive malignant melanoma with the potential to produce distant metastases. The less common nodular melanoma will show abnormal melanocytes extending into the dermis producing a nodular tumour without extension into the surrounding epidermis. Often, but not inevitably, there is a lymphocytic infiltrate at the edge of the tumour. Tumours may show variable amounts of melanin, and if there is doubt about the type of pigmentation then special stains may be useful such as S^{100} and HMB-45. Secondary deposits of malignant melanoma may look very similar but will not have any direct link with the epidermis and are usually entirely dermal.

THE CLARK LEVEL OF INVASION AND BRESLOW THICKNESS

Both of these are a measurement of the depth of invasion, the single most important indicator of prognosis and the most important part of the pathology report after establishing the diagnosis. Clark recognized that

Table 4.1
Clark level of invasion.

Level
1 Intraepidermal (*in situ*)
2 Papillary dermis by single cells
3 Upper dermis
4 Reticular dermis
5 Subcutaneous fat

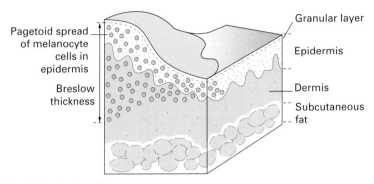

Pagetoid spread of melanocyte cells in epidermis

Breslow thickness

Granular layer

Epidermis

Dermis

Subcutaneous fat

Fig. 4.1 The Breslow thickness.

there was a relationship between the level of invasion of the tumour and the ultimate prognosis [2]. He divided the levels of invasion into five separate levels (Table 4.1).

Breslow refined this and demonstrated that a direct measurement of the tumour thickness, measured in millimetres, from the granular layer to the deepest abnormal tumour cell (Fig. 4.1), gave a very good indicator of prognosis at five years and the likelihood of metastatic spread (Table 4.2) [3]. Usually, the Breslow thickness and the Clark level of invasion coincide. Occasionally, for instance if the epidermis is very thin, the tumour may have a narrow Breslow thickness but a deeper Clark level of invasion. In general it is easier to concentrate on the Breslow thickness and to use this as the main measure of predicting prognosis and planning further management. Patients with lesions that are less than 0.75 mm in depth have a five-year survival rate approaching 100%. There is then a gradually worsening

Breslow thickness (mm)	Surviving 5 years (%)
Intraepidermal	100
< 0.75	98
0.75–1.5	85
1.5–4.00	70
> 4.00	45

Table 4.2
5-Year survival rates according to Breslow thickness.

Breslow thickness	Years					
	1	2	3	4	5	6–10
< 1mm	1.2	0.8	1.6	0	0.6	0.3
1–3.5 mm	6.3	9.7	6.8	3.1	2.9	1.5
3.5 mm +	32	25	14	12.5	2	3.5

Table 4.3
Percentage of patients with primary malignant melanoma who develop recurrence each year according to Breslow thickness [4].

picture, so those patients presenting with lesions greater than 4 mm in depth have about a 30% chance of surviving five years (Table 4.3). These predictions are the same regardless of the site of the tumour, type of tumour, sex or other variables. The Breslow thickness is the main measurement used in planning further surgical treatment (see Chapter 5).

Other histopathological indicators of prognosis

The terms 'horizontal growth phase' and 'vertical growth phase' give an indication as to the pattern of spread of the melanoma cells. If the growth phase is horizontal, this means that the tumour is mainly confined to the epidermis and junctional layer of the epidermis and extends only minimally into the dermis. This implies a good prognosis tumour. A vertical growth phase implies that the lesion is invading dermally and the prognosis will therefore be worse.

Ulceration is a poor prognostic sign which is usually obvious macroscopically, but occasionally may be microscopic only. Similarly, if there is vascular invasion with tumour cells within blood vessels in the dermis, this indicates that the patient will have a worse prognosis than that indicated on the Breslow thickness alone.

The pathologist may mention the presence of regression. Regression implies that there has been an immune reaction against the tumour with a marked lymphocytic infiltration sometimes seen. The tumour may have been thicker than the current measurement on the Breslow scale implies, and therefore may indicate a worse prognosis. A high number of mitoses is also a bad sign which the pathologist may comment on and may give the actual number seen per high power field.

All of these features aid the clinician in making an overall estimate of the prognosis for the individual patients. Indeed, there are computer programmes now available into which many of these features can be entered giving a five-year survival rate based on all the factors which are known to affect survival. For most clinicians however, the single most important indicator continues to be the Breslow thickness, which far overrides any of the other prognostic indicators.

THE NATURAL HISTORY OF MALIGNANT MELANOMA

It is, of course, impossible to observe the natural history of melanoma as they are all removed as soon as they are diagnosed. There is some controversy as to whether or not some of the very early tumours, which are now seen commonly, would ever progress to a frankly malignant tumour if left alone. Simply observing these tumours would, however, be unethical.

There are several studies which give a good indication of the natural history of melanoma, based on analysis of the time taken to the development of metastatic disease and death related to Breslow thickness at presentation. The annual risk of recurrence or development of metastases of a malignant melanoma are shown in Table 4.2. The risk depends on the depth of the lesion. Lesions which are entirely intra-epidermal have no potential for metastatic spread. Patients with thin lesions (< 1 mm in depth) have an approximate 1% chance of recurrence per annum for the first three years, reducing down to 0.3% per annum after five years. This contrasts with patients with thicker lesions (> 3.5 mm in depth), where almost a third will develop a recurrence within the first 12 months and 70% within the first three years [4].

REFERENCES

1 Mackie RM. Malignant melanoma. In: Champion R, Burton J, Burns A, Breathnach S. eds. *Textbook of Dermatology*, 6th edn. Blackwell Science, 1998; 1740–3.

2 Clark WH, Jnr, Ainsworth AM, Bernandino EA. The developmental biology of primary human malignant melanomas. *Semin Oncol* 1975; **2**: 83–103.

3 Breslow A. Thickness, cross-sectional area and depth of invasion in the prognosis of cutaneous melanoma. *Ann Surg* 1970; **172**: 902–8.

4 Dicker TJ *et al*. A rational approach to melanoma follow-up in patients with primary cutaneous melanoma. *Br J Derm* 1999; **140**: 249–54.

5 Surgery: No Margin for Error

The management of primary cutaneous malignant melanoma is entirely surgical and is deceptively simple. It has changed greatly over the last 20 years, as the margins of excision have become progressively narrower as a result of a better understanding of the behaviour of the disease. Up until the late 1970s the margins advised were often 4–5 inches around the tumour. This resulted in people having disfiguring excisions for what were, at times, very thin tumours. The work of Clark and Breslow in the late 1960s and 1970s established that the thickness of the tumour at the time of excision was of great prognostic importance and that thin tumours were far less likely to spread than thick tumours (see Chapter 4). This was followed by a small series of clinical trials on excision margins, which have confirmed that the large excision margins of the past are no longer necessary and that patients do just as well with narrower margins. This has completely changed the management of malignant melanoma. About 70% of patients now present with thin lesions, which can usually be easily managed with a local anaesthetic in an outpatient or day care setting.

SURGICAL MANAGEMENT OF SUSPICIOUS LESIONS

The clinical diagnosis of malignant melanoma can be very difficult, and any pigmented lesion which looks suspicious, or which has changed in the recent past, should be excised in total for histological diagnosis. This can almost always be carried out under local anaesthetic and the lesion should be removed with a clear 2–3 mm margin. Patients with clinically obvious malignant melanomas can be dealt with in the same way. This allows confirmation of the diagnosis histologically and allows the surgeon to plan the definitive margin of excision once the Breslow thickness is available (Table 5.1). If at all possible the lesion should be excised completely. Incisional biopsies are not usually recommended because the biopsy taken may not be fully representative and both diagnosis and measurement of the depth of invasion may be difficult. Although there is a theoretical risk of dissemination of the tumour if the tumour is incised rather than completely

Breslow thickness	Surgical excision margins
Intra-epidermal	Clear histological margins
< 1 mm	1 cm
1–2 mm	1–2 cm
2–4 mm	2 cm
4 mm	2–3 cm

Table 5.1
Surgical excision margins for malignant melanoma according to Breslow thickness.

removed, in practice this has never been proven to be the case. Incisional diagnostic biopsies can sometimes be justified when it would be difficult to excise the lesion in full or because of the size or site of the lesion. For instance, in a suspected lentigo maligna melanoma of the face, covering a large area, the thicker part of the tumour could be biopsied. If the clinical diagnosis is clear, then some surgeons prefer to excise the lesion in full, with a 1 cm margin, which saves the patient having two operative procedures.

DEFINITIVE SURGERY

Once the pathology report comes through it should be read carefully, taking into account, in particular, the surgical margins of excision of the primary tumour, as reported both macroscopically and microscopically, and the Breslow thickness (Chapter 4). The Breslow thickness is the single most important indicator of prognosis and the definitive surgical margins will be based on the thickness of the tumour. There are no studies on the most appropriate depth of excision. Most surgeons now excise through the subcutaneous fat to the underlying fascia but not through the fascia itself.

Intra-epidermal melanoma *in situ* or lentigo maligna

These have no potential for metastatic spread and the aim of surgery is simply to excise the lesion in total with a clear histological margin. No further treatment is then required.

Lesions less than 1 mm in depth

The margins recommended for these lesions are based on a trial reported in 1991 [1]. This was a landmark trial which compared the recurrence rate of melanomas treated with either a 1 cm or a 3 cm margin. In patients with lesions less than 1 mm thick there were no recurrences with either excision margin. It was therefore firmly concluded that a 1 cm margin of excision was safe and appropriate for these lesions. Most of these can be removed with a local anaesthetic. The margin around the lesion or the excisional scar is measured to 1 cm on either side and the lesion is then formally excised. The wound can usually be repaired leaving a neat linear scar.

Lesions 1–2 mm in depth

The margins recommended are based on two large randomized studies. The first study showed no difference in overall survival, between patients having 1 and 3 cm margins. However, a small number developed local recurrences as the first sign of relapse, all of whom had undergone excision with a 1 cm margin. The authors were therefore cautious in recommending 1 cm margins for this group, and suggested that 2 cm margins may be more appropriate [1]. The Intergroup Melanoma trial compared 2 versus 4 cm margins of excision for lesions 1–4 mm in depth, and showed that there was no difference in the local recurrence rate or survival in these patients. The authors suggested, therefore, that margins greater than 2 cm are inappropriate for this group [2]. Most authorities recommend a margin of between 1 and 2 cm for these patients, and certainly margins greater than this are not necessary.

Lesions 2–4 mm in depth

On the basis of the Intergroup Melanoma trial, it has been shown that there is no difference between 2 cm and 4 cm margins for patients in this group in either overall survival or recurrence rates [2], and most authorities would recommend 2 cm margins wherever possible for patients with these deeper tumours.

Lesions greater than 4 mm in depth

Patients with lesions greater than 4 mm in depth have a poor prognosis. These patients have never been included in any randomized studies. It has been recognized for many years that patients in this group have a high incidence of local recurrences if the margins are too narrow, and patients should therefore have the lesions excised with a 2–3 cm margin. Patients

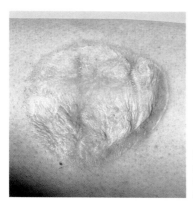

Fig. 5.1
A typical skin graft following
removal of a melanoma with
a 3 cm margin.

having margins of 2–3 cm often have to have the wounds repaired with skin
grafts, but this will depend on the anatomical site (Fig. 5.1).

OTHER TREATMENTS

Cryotherapy is occasionally used for patients with lentigo maligna and
can give good cosmetic results. Elderly, infirm patients with superficially
invasive lentigo maligna melanoma can also be treated in this way, but the
risk of recurrence is high and long-term surveillance is necessary (Fig. 5.2).

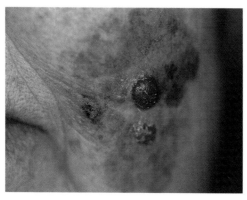

Fig. 5.2
Recurrence of a lentigo
maligna melanoma following
treatment with cryotherapy.

Radiotherapy is sometimes used as a primary treatment for patients with lentigo maligna melanoma who are not suitable for surgery.

LYMPH NODE DISSECTION

Elective lymph node dissection

Elective lymph node dissection means the removal of clinically non-affected lymph nodes from the area draining the tumour. For instance, patients with a melanoma on their arm would have a full axillary clearance, whereas those with tumours on the leg would have their inguinal nodes dissected. Some specialists are keen advocates of elective lymph node dissection, however, the two prospective randomized studies that have been carried out showed no improvement in survival in patients treated in this way [3,4]. The studies have been criticized and the topic is still controversial. New techniques are currently being developed to identify 'sentinel nodes'. Sentinel nodes can be identified in more than 80% of patients by injecting a blue dye intradermally around the tumour or by means of intraoperative gamma probes. Biopsy of the sentinel node can accurately predict if any of the other lymph nodes are involved in 95% of patients. This technique is not in routine use as yet, and is still under investigation [5].

Therapeutic lymph node dissection

This is used when there is clinical evidence that the glands draining the affected area are involved. Removing the lymph nodes in that area gives a longer, disease free survival.

REFERENCES

1 Veronesi U, Cascinelli N. Narrow excision (1 cm margin): a safe procedure for thin cutaneous melanoma. *Arch Surg* 1991; **126**: 438–41.

2 Balch CM, Urist MM, Karakousis CP *et al.* Efficacy of 2 cm surgical margins for intermediate—thickness melanomas (1–4 mm): result of a multi-institutional randomised surgical trial. *Ann Surg* 1993; **218**: 262–7.

3 Sim FH, Taylor WF, Pritchard DJ *et al.* Lymphadenectomy in the management of stage 1 malignant melanoma: a prospective randomised study. *Mayo Clin Proc* 1986; **61**: 697–705.

4 Veronesi U, Adams J, Bandiera DC *et al*. Delayed regional lymph node dissection in stage 1 malignant melanoma of the skin of the lower extremities. *Cancer* 1982; **49**: 2420–30.

5 Rivers RK, Roof MI. Sentinel lymph-node biopsy in melanoma: is less surgery better? *Lancet*, 1997; **350**: 1336–7.

6 Follow-up: What Happens Now?

TALKING ABOUT THE DIAGNOSIS

Few diseases are associated with such fear and dread as cancer. Many patients these days are aware that skin cancer does not lead to early death in most cases, however, the term malignant melanoma is frightening and can conjure up images of pain, suffering and certain death. The challenge for the physician is to help the patient to understand the diagnosis and set the disease in context, explaining the treatment, future management and prognosis in a caring and considerate manner.

Many patients when they first present to a doctor with a change in a pigmented lesion do not seriously believe that they have a type of skin cancer as there is still a perception that all cancers are painful and, in particular with melanoma, that all malignant lesions itch or bleed. The diagnosis of a malignant melanoma may therefore come as a surprise to many patients, and the possibility should be suggested to them in a gentle, considered manner as they may feel overwhelmed by the diagnosis and by any subsequent information given to them. It is useful to try to assess the attitude of the patient before the diagnosis is given. During the initial consultation when the physician is suspicious that the lesion may be a malignant melanoma, it may be quite useful to ask patients questions such as 'What do you think this may be?' 'Have you thought of the possibility that this could be a type of skin cancer?' or 'Have you any particular anxieties as to what may be causing these changes?' The patient may then be prepared gently and in stages for the possibility that the lesion may turn out to be a malignant melanoma. At the next consultation following excision of the lesion, if the diagnosis is confirmed, once again the clinician will have to be cautious and considerate in imparting the diagnosis to the patient. It is important to allow the patient sufficient time to take in the diagnosis and its implications, and there must be enough opportunity for the patient to ask questions.

If the melanoma is a thin lesion with a good prognosis it is usually easy to reassure the patient but some patients will be so shocked by the fact

39

that they have had a cancer that they will remember very little of the reassurances and will walk out of the consultation room in a daze. In this situation, if possible, a nurse should be available to sit down with the patient to discuss and explain matters further, and the general practitioner should receive information about the diagnosis as soon as possible. Some patients, particularly the elderly and those that have a good relationship with their family doctor, will wish to discuss the diagnosis and receive support in this way at an early stage.

Many patients believe that all cancers are lethal and will be surprised to learn that most patients with malignant melanoma are completely cured. During the initial consultation the patient should not be overloaded with information, as they will inevitably forget a great deal of what has been said. The patient will need to be seen regularly by both the specialist and general practitioner and further information can be given in stages and, if necessary, the same information repeated. The patient should be asked from time to time if they understand what has been said to them, and if there are any questions that they would like to ask. The patient should also be reassured that if they are concerned in any way about their condition, that there is an open door policy, both with the general practitioner and in the specialist unit. The best departments will give a direct line telephone number that patients can ring and arrange appointments to be seen by the specialist within a few days. Written information, as a back up to the information already given verbally, should be given to all patients. The written information should be clear and unambiguous and should contain telephone numbers of medical or nursing staff who can be contacted if they are concerned. Communication between primary care and secondary care is vital if the patient is to maintain confidence in their medical helpers. Specialists should ensure that general practitioners receive information about the diagnosis and prognosis within a day or two of the diagnosis being made, and the general practitioner should feel free to discuss the details of the management with the specialist at any time.

THE PATIENT'S EDUCATION

After the initial consultations and discussion with the patient about the diagnosis and immediate management, over the next few weeks the emphasis should be on patient education. Advice on future sun exposure should be given so that the patient is reminded to avoid sunburn and excessive sun exposure with the help of clothing, hats and sunscreen. I believe that it is important not to be too judgemental with regard to the possibility that previous sun exposure has been excessive and may have caused the skin cancer, as it is difficult enough to cope with the fact that one has developed a melanoma, and making a patient feel guilty about their past behaviour in the sun is unhelpful. The patient can be instructed on self-examination and information provided on the changes which they should look out for in other moles which they may have. This is particularly true for patients with multiple naevi or those with dysplastic naevi and they should be given clear, concise advice and told to report immediately any changes in size, shape or colour of any existing moles. They should also be shown how to examine their regional lymph glands. Most patients are ready and willing to accept this and do not become overtly anxious about doing so. Written information can, again, be very useful to support what is told to patients in consulting rooms.

HOSPITAL FOLLOW-UP

All patients with invasive malignant melanoma will be followed up in a specialist department over a period of years. The reasons for following patients up are both to educate them and to detect recurrences and new primary lesions. There is no agreed protocol for follow-up but most specialists will tend to follow-up patients three monthly for the first year or two and then six monthly for a total of about five years. Patients may be followed up longer if there are particular reasons, such as the development of a second primary, or if the patient has multiple dysplastic naevi. On each follow-up visit, patients will have the initial scar examined as, particularly with thick lesions, the first sign of metastatic disease may occur around the primary scar. The regional lymph nodes will be carefully examined, and a full body examination paying particular attention to other pigmented lesions will be carried out.

The patient's concerns can be discussed and the doctor can reinforce previous advice on self-examination, sun awareness and recognition of other abnormal pigmented lesions. The risk of recurrence or metastases of a malignant melanoma are shown in Table 4.3 (page 30). The risk depends on the depth of the lesion. Lesions which are entirely intraepidermal have no potential for metastatic spread. Patients with thin lesions (> 1 mm in depth) have an approximate 1% chance of recurrence per annum for the first three years, reducing down to 0.3% per annum after five years. This contrasts with patients with thicker lesions (< 3.5 mm in depth), where almost a third will develop a recurrence within the first 12 months and 70% within the first three years [1].

SUPPORT

All patients will need support following the diagnosis of malignant melanoma. This may be provided by friends and family and supported to varying degrees by health professionals. The type of support provided will depend on the patient and the facilities available. Many cancer centres employ professional counsellors who may be able to give advice and general support, as well as specialist nurses who can be invaluable in this situation. The primary health care team, who may know the patients very well, are often in a better position than hospital specialist departments in helping patients through what can be a very difficult period. There are also established charities, both local and national, which can provide support through telephone helplines and written information.

REFERENCE

1 Dicker TJ *et al.* A rational approach to melanoma follow-up in patients with primary cutaneous melanoma. *Br J Derm* 1999; **140**: 249–54.

7 Second Line Therapies: What Happens Next?

It must be emphasized that most patients with malignant melanoma are treated entirely by surgery. However, several other treatments are available for those with recurrent and metastatic disease. Once metastases occur, whether this is localized or systemic, the prognosis is altered dramatically. Successful treatment is most likely when the disease remains localized around the original scar or when only the regional lymph nodes are involved. Once the metastases spread elsewhere in the body, treatment has only little to offer. The most that the majority of patients with secondaries can hope for is an extension of life by a few weeks or months, rather than a complete remission (Fig. 7.1).

SURGERY

Most patients who develop secondaries usually present with recurrent lesions around the site of the original scar or in the regional lymph nodes. Surgery is the best option for treatment at this stage. For cutaneous secondaries occurring either around the scar or between the site of the original excision scar and the regional lymph nodes, surgical excision is the best option for treatment. They can usually be easily excised with a local anaesthetic if they are not too numerous.

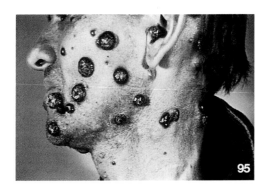

Fig. 7.1
Metastatic malignant melanoma.

Involvement of regional lymph nodes may be determined clinically by palpation or following a sentinel node biopsy (see Chapter 5). If a lymph node is suspected of being involved, the surgeon will usually take a biopsy. If this is confirmed as being affected the surgeon will then progress to a full therapeutic lymph node dissection removing all of the lymph nodes in the draining area. This can be complicated and difficult and does have quite a high morbidity. Chronic lymphoedema of a limb is commonplace afterwards. However, there is no doubt that removal of affected lymph nodes, if this is the only site of metastatic spread, can have a beneficial effect on prognosis.

ISOLATED LIMB PERFUSION

This is a highly specialized technique used for treating multiple cutaneous metastatic lesions in a limb, when there is no evidence of spread elsewhere. This technique is only carried out in a few specialist centres. The limb, usually the leg, is isolated from the rest of the arterial circulation under general anaesthetic and perfused with a chemotherapeutic agent (usually Melphalan). Often the cutaneous lesions regress following this treatment, but there is no guarantee that this will improve long-term survival. The technique is difficult and time consuming and can have a high morbidity, but can be useful in selected patients, as it can prolong disease free survival in some individuals.

LASER TREATMENTS

Lasers in general do not have a large part to play in the treatment of melanoma. The CO_2 laser in cutting mode has been used successfully in excising cutaneous lesions when these are multiple but this, in reality, offers little benefit over conventional excisional surgery.

CHEMOTHERAPY

Chemotherapy is used when there is evidence of systemic metastases, particularly when these are at sites which are difficult to excise surgically. A variety of combinations of different chemotherapeutic agents have been tried, but the most reliable results are obtained with DTIC (Dacarbazine), which can be used either alone or in combination. The results of treatment are often disappointing but may prolong life for an extra few weeks or months. It is important to discuss this with the patient in some detail as the extension of life may be at the expense of quality of life. Treatment with chemotherapy should only be carried out by a qualified oncologist, and anyone with metastatic disease should have the benefit of a consultation with an oncologist with an interest in melanoma.

RADIOTHERAPY

Malignant melanoma is usually regarded as a radio resistant tumour, but occasionally radiotherapy can be useful in the treatment of isolated internal metastatic lesions. Radiotherapy can also be used in relieving the pain of bony secondaries. Occasionally radiotherapy can be used as a primary treatment for the management of elderly patients with lentigo maligna melanoma when these patients are considered to be unsuitable for treatment with surgery, usually because they are elderly and very infirm and the tumour covers a large area of skin.

INTERFERON

Interferons are currently being intensively investigated in large international clinical trials, and their place in management of melanoma is not yet clear. There seems little doubt that their use has an appreciable effect on the biology and progression of melanoma. However, there is no agreement as yet on the correct dosage and the stage at which they are best utilized. Interferons have been used in different ways. A recent study of high dose Interferon in patients with high risk tumours did show some improvement in survival, but this was at the expense of toxicity and quality of life. The treatment is also very expensive. Low dose Interferon treatment which is far less toxic has also been used, and there is some evidence that the use of low dose Interferons in melanomas which are only moderately thick (1.5 mm plus) may give some benefit to survival. There seems little doubt that Interferons do have a part to play in the management of patients with melanoma, but further trials are needed before they can be recommended for routine use. Hopefully, as the new trials currently underway progress, their role will become clearer. It is certainly worthwhile considering anyone with a moderate to thick melanoma for adjuvant treatment with Interferons and these patients should be reviewed in a specialist centre and, if possible, entered into one of the current trials [1].

VACCINES

Unlike the use of vaccines for the prevention of infectious diseases, vaccines for melanoma are being developed as a therapeutic agent for patients with metastatic disease. Several types of vaccines are currently being investigated alone and in combination with other therapies such as Interferons. Melanomas do seem to be susceptible to this type of treatment and initial studies have been encouraging. Vaccines are not currently available for routine therapeutic use however, and patients can only obtain vaccine treatment by being enrolled into one of the current trials [2].

PALLIATIVE CARE

It is important to involve the palliative care team at an early stage in any patient who has evidence of metastatic spread, whether this be local or systemic. The palliative care team will have expertise in the management of patients with advanced cancers and will be able to support the patient emotionally and physically through their illness. There are several advances in the management of chronic pain which the palliative care consultant will be able to advise on. Nurses and counsellors attached to the palliative care team will be able to support the patient and family, both in hospital and at home, and will play an increasingly important role in helping the patient as the disease progresses.

REFERENCES

1 Agarwala SS, Kirkwood JM. Adjuvant therapy of melanoma. *Semin Surg Oncol* 1998; **14**: 4: 302–10.
2 Ollila DW, Kelley MC, Gammon G, Morton DL. Overview of melanoma vaccines: active specific immunotherapy for melanoma patients. *Semin Surg Onol* 1998; **14**: 4: 328–36.

8 Prevention and Early Detection: Theory and Practice

THE CHALLENGE

Can the numbers of new melanomas and the death toll from established melanoma be reduced?

Two thirds of all melanomas are attributed to excessive sun exposure; reducing this should result in a decline in the numbers of new cases (primary prevention). Detection and treatment of early melanomas could significantly reduce the mortality rate as thin melanomas carry a much better prognosis than thicker lesions (secondary prevention). That is the theory but, in practice, it is not that simple.

PRIMARY PREVENTION

Since the 1930s many white people have regarded the acquisition of a suntan as desirable, signifying not only health but also wealth and beauty. Increased levels of sun exposure, particularly the episodic exposure of fair skin, remains the most significant factor in the development of melanoma. Other recognized risk factors include the presence of atypical naevi, large numbers of benign pigmented naevi, skin types 1 or 2 and having blonde or red hair (see Chapter 1).

Advising patients to follow simple guidelines could reduce the overall level of sun exposure. These can be summarized as:

1 minimize sun exposure around midday;

2 seek the shade;

3 wear protective clothing; and

4 correctly use a sunscreen with a sun protection factor (SPF) of 15 or higher.

UVB peaks between the hours of 11am and 3pm, especially in the summer months. Clouds block very little UV radiation and swimming offers little protection as UV can penetrate the water surface. Natural shade, such as trees, gives good protection. UV is reflected from snow and sand but less so from grassy surfaces. A wide brimmed hat can shade the face and neck and closely woven dark clothes and sunglasses also provide good personal shade.

The use of sunscreens is complementary to the above. Sunscreens should be applied to prevent excessive sun exposure rather than prolong it. There is no hard evidence to prove that they prevent melanoma but the assumption that they can help is a reasonable one [1]. Modern preparations protect against both UVB and UVA. The sun protection factor (SPF) is a measure of the ability to protect against UVB. For example, an SPF of 15 should enable a person to remain 15 times longer in the sun without burning. Few are correctly applied and the protection achieved is typically only 20–50%. UVA protection is measured by star rating of 1–4 with 4 being the strongest. Four stars indicate protection equal to that of the UVB protection. The efficacy of sunscreens depends on other factors including the thickness and frequency of application, sweating, bathing and the strength of the sun.

CHANGING BEHAVIOUR

How and why people's behaviour changes are both complex and poorly understood. One theory that has been successfully applied to a number of health-related issues views change as a gradual process involving several stages. Individuals may move from a stage where they are not interested in change to a stage where change is contemplated and then progress to actually making a change. Tailoring the approach to the individual's stage on the road to sun protection may produce more effective results [2].

Children

Babies and small children are extremely vulnerable. Their skin should be protected from strong sunlight at all times. Parents and/or other carers should be encouraged to provide adequate protection such as shade, clothing and sunscreens. Sun awareness education should begin in the antenatal period and continue through preschool and school. A 'sun-aware' child may grow up to be a more responsible adult.

Teenagers

On average more than half the lifetime UV exposure occurs before adulthood but modification of any teenage behaviour is not easy. As well as education, behaviour may be influenced by role models such as beach lifeguards and sports personalities. Appearance is important and teenagers may be more influenced by the fact that excessive sun exposure prematurely ages the skin rather than the long term risks of skin cancer. There is a welcome trend in some fashion and teen magazines towards less tanned models and increased information on sun protection [3]. There is scope for more active media involvement, especially that aimed at young men.

Adults

A targeted approach to the adult population may be more cost-effective. For example, in many countries, outdoor workers have become a specific target of national campaigns. At a primary care level it would be possible to identify other groups at higher risk such as holidaymakers requesting travel advice, those with fair skin (types 1 and 2) or those with a history of sunburn [4].

The local community

Towns and neighbourhoods should be encouraged to provide shade in public places especially children's play areas. Does your neighbourhood school have a policy on sun protection? Local communities should also be encouraged to participate in national campaigns.

At a national level

Many countries produce high quality sun awareness campaigns. The primary and secondary care health providers should be active participants in these. Some are now available on the Internet [5]. Several countries incorporate sun warnings into their weather reports.

At a global level

The international community has reached some agreement to decrease stratospheric ozone depletion in particular by eliminating the use of chlorofluorocarbons (CFCs). Although over 50 countries ratified the Montreal Protocol (1987) there are some notable exceptions who continue to manufacture and use CFCs.

EVALUATION OF PRIMARY PROTECTION

The ultimate aims are to achieve a fall in the incidence of and mortality from melanoma. Because there is a latent period of several decades between sun exposure and melanoma development the effects of most campaigns have not been fully evaluated. A number of intermediate outcome measures have been proposed. These include improved attitudes to sun awareness with greater use of protective clothing and sunscreens and decreased rates of sunburn and deliberate sunbathing. The Sunsmart campaign has been running in Australia for several years. With its theme of 'Slip!Slop!Slap!' (slip on a shirt, slop on a sunscreen and slap on a hat) there has been a significant change in attitude and behaviour [6].

SECONDARY PREVENTION

The early detection and treatment of thin melanomas can save lives. Early detection ranges from the casual self-examination by the average risk individual to the very regular entire skin examination by a specialist in skin cancer. Melanomas are by and large visible and their features recognizable. However the preoperative diagnostic accuracy of specialist dermatologists may be only around 70%. Programmes designed to inform the public of the features of early melanoma must be easily understood but sensitive enough to pick up most malignant lesions. Inevitably this will lead to the reporting of a large number of benign lesions such as pigmented naevi and seborrhoeic warts. Not only is there a need for greater public education but also for all doctors and other health care professionals who may be consulted regarding a 'suspicious' lesion. Success of any campaign depends on wide publicity involving both the press and the television. The resultant increase in workload must be planned for carefully. There needs to be increased training at primary care level, sufficient specialist services (e.g. dermatologists and plastic surgeons) that can be rapidly accessed and fast, accurate pathological services.

EVALUATION OF SECONDARY PREVENTION

Unlike primary prevention campaigns, the effect of early detection should be apparent in a few years. A fall in the absolute numbers of thick melanomas and a decrease in the mortality rate would indicate a successful campaign. These measures rely on very accurate data recording both before and after any campaign. Not all activities have been carefully audited but there is an overall impression that early detection campaigns have led to the presentation of melanomas at an earlier stage. In the west of Scotland, where there is a high incidence of melanoma, intensive public education and early detection activities have resulted in a fall in the mortality in women [7].

CONCLUSION

Reducing the burden of malignant melanoma relies heavily on successful primary prevention and early detection. Campaigns are now being carried out in numerous countries. It is essential that these are carefully audited and that the most effective ways of achieving their goals are identified. There is evidence to indicate that knowledge with regard to sun exposure is improving but there is less evidence that actual behaviour is changing. If the challenge of melanoma is to be met then future campaigns must determine and implement the most effective methods of prevention and early detection.

REFERENCES

1 Anonymous. Do sunscreens prevent skin cancer. *Drug Ther Bull* 1998; **36**: 7: 49–51.
2 Prochaska JO. Assessing how people change. *Cancer* 1991; **67**: 805–7.
3 George PM, Kuskowski M. Trends in photoprotection in American fashion magazines, 1983–93. *J Am Acad Dermatol* 1996; **34**: 3: 424–8.
4 Jackson A, Wilkinson C, Ranger M, Pill R, August P. Can primary prevention or selective screening for melanoma be more precisely targeted through general practice? A prospective study to validate a self administered risk score. *BMJ* 1998; **316**: 34–9.
5 www.melanomanet.com.
6 Hill D, White V, Marks R, Borland R. Changes in sun-related attitudes and behaviour, and reduced sunburn prevalence in a population at high risk of melanoma. *Eur J Cancer Prev* 1993; **2**: 6: 447–56.
7 MacKie RM, Hole D. Audit of public education campaign to encourage earlier detection of malignant melanoma. *BMJ* 1992; **304**: 1012–15.

FURTHER READING

1 Koh HK, Geller AC. Public health interventions for melanoma. Prevention, early detection, and education. *Hematol Oncol Clin North Am* 1998; **12**: 4: 903–28.
2 MacKie RM. Melanoma prevention and early detection. *Br Med Bull* 1995; **51**: 3: 570–83.

Index

Page numbers in *italics* refer to picture captions; those in **bold** refer to tables.